I0844187

REVERSE HIGH BLOOD PRESSURE

Healthy Recipes

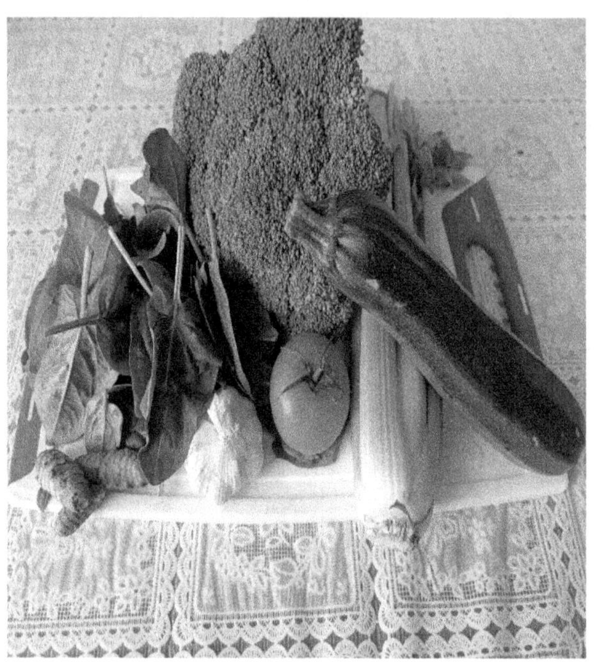

Introduction

This book is going to explain how I control my blood pressure based on my personal experience after I was diagnosed in 2016.

I am not a Physician nor a Doctor or Medical adviser but I will share my experience with you. I was consistent in keeping my blood pressure under control.

this book i will show you the most powerful hypertension-crushing recipes you will find
nywhere
igh blood pressure, also known as hypertension, is a medical condition in which the
rce of blood against the walls of the arteries is consistently too high. It is a common
ealth problem that affects millions of people worldwide.
igh blood pressure, the heart exerts pressure to pump blood in the body.
s normal pressure is considered to be 120/80 mm of mercury.
 hypertension this pressure stays higher than the normal limit
was able to reduce my blood pressure from 180/110 mm of mercury
  121/78 mm of mercury.
igh blood pressure leads to strain on heart conditions like kidney failure and stroke.

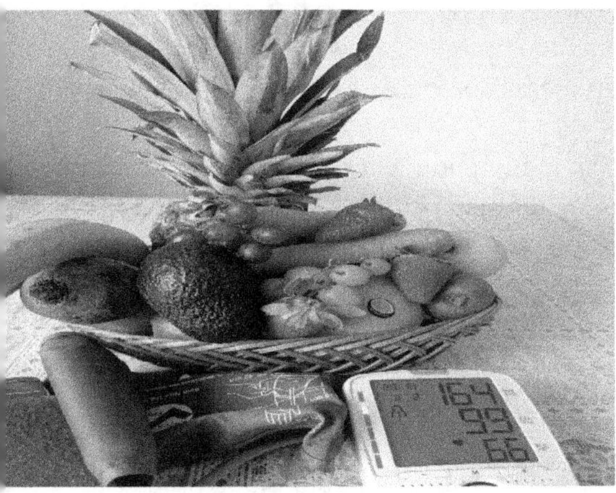

alcium rich food to reduce high blood pressure
ontracts & dilates heart muscles makes blood flow smoother, Milk, Tofu, Yogurt
otassium rich food that reduce High blood pressure
alances excess water in body, lowers blood pressure
mega 3, improves blood circulation eg. Fish, Flaxseeds, Coconut water, Bananas,
ates,Oranges, Pomegranate, Figs, Mangoes, Watermelon, Broccoli, tomatoes,
eetroot and Bell peppers.
agnesium rich food that reduces high blood pressure Relaxes muscles that control
ood vessels. Almonds, Walnut, Barley, Spinach, Pumpkin seeds, Sunflower

High Blood Pressure

ypertension measure

here are two main types of hypertension:
rimary (essential) hypertension: This is the most common type and develops gradually
ver time with no identifiable cause. It is usually related to a combination of genetic
ctors, lifestyle choices, and age-related changes.

Secondary hypertension: This type of high blood pressure is caused by an underlying medical condition or medication. It usually appears suddenly and tends to be more severe than primary hypertension. Some conditions that can lead to secondary hypertension include kidney disease, hormonal disorders, certain medications, and sleep apnea.

Managing high blood pressure involves a combination of lifestyle modifications and, in some cases, medication. Here are some strategies to help control blood pressure: Healthy regular exercise: Engage in physical activity for at least 150 minutes per week. can include brisk walking, jogging, swimming, cycling, or any other aerobic exercise.Weight management: Maintain a healthy weight or work towards achieving a healthy weight if overweight. Losing even a small amount of weight can significantly lower blood pressure.

Limit alcohol consumption: Drink alcohol in moderation. Limiting intake to one drink per day for women and up to two drinks per day for men is generally recommended.

Quit smoking: Smoking can raise your blood pressure and damage your blood vessels. Quitting smoking is essential for overall cardiovascular health.

Reduce stress: Find healthy ways to manage stress, such as practicing relaxation techniques, exercising, engaging in hobbies, or seeking support from friends and family.

Medication: Depending on the severity of high blood pressure, your doctor may prescribe medication to help lower and control your blood pressure. It's important to take the prescribed medication as directed and regularly monitor your blood pressure.

Regular check-ups with a healthcare professional are important to monitor your blood pressure and make any necessary adjustments to your treatment plan. By adopting a healthy lifestyle and following medical advice, many people can effectively manage their blood pressure and reduce the risk of associated complication

Visit us at: https://www.digistore24.com/redir/447648/IsaacAustin/

Chapter 1

BREAKFAST

Before breakfast:

30 minutes before breakfast take a glass of water with lemon juice (self pressed) add a half teaspoon of Honey. Take a little exercise for some few minutes between 10-20 minutes

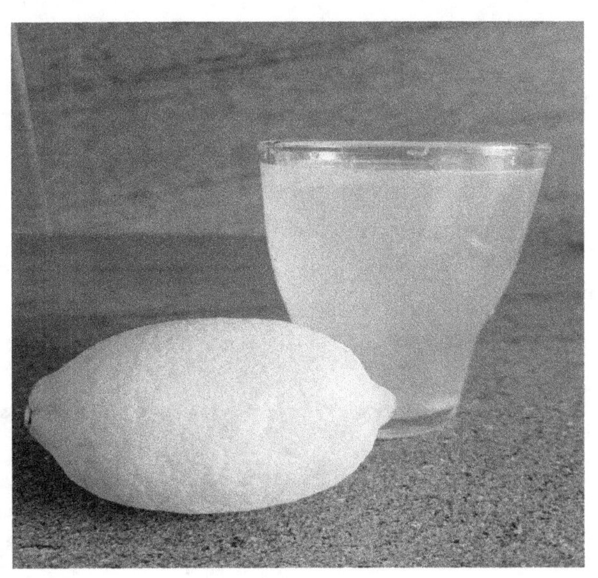

arm water, lemon and honey

Chapter 2

Breakfast / Porridge with Berries

Recipe 1

Ingredients:

1: 1.5 Cups unsweetened almond milk
2: 1/3 cup shredded coconut
3: 3 tablespoons almond meal
4: 2 tablespoon ground flaxseed
5. 3/4 cup mix of blueberries, blackberries and coarsely chopped strawberries
6: 2 tablespoon toasted pecans
7: 3 pieces of Dates(chopped)

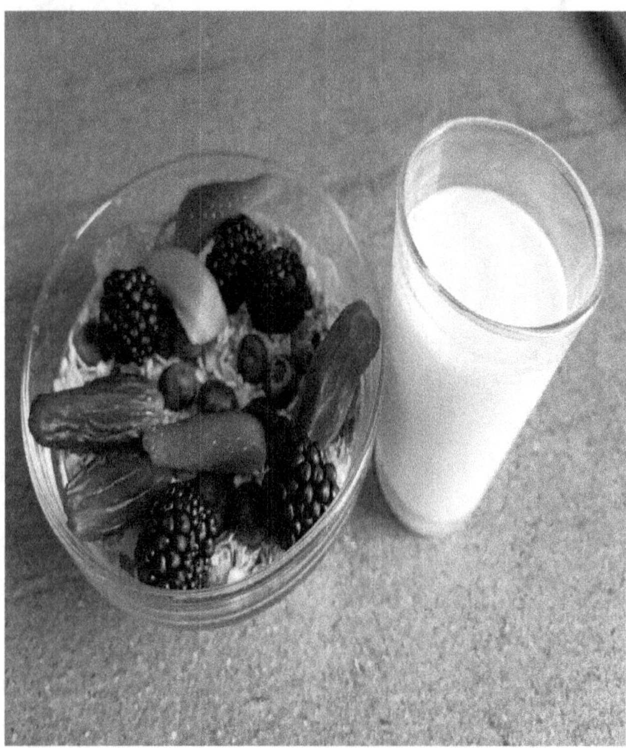

Steps:

1) Heat the almond milk on a medium-low heat
2) Stir the ingredients aside from the berries once the mixture starts to simme
3) Cook the mixture for 1 minute
4) Place the mixture into two bowls. Top with berries and toasted pecans

Chapter 3

Breakfast / Yogurt with fruits

Recipe 2

Ingredients:

1: 250g of low fat Yogurt
2: Handful of Almond
3: 1 Banane 1 Apfel
4: 1 Teaspoon of Cinnamon
5: Handful of mix blueberries, blackberries
6: Handful of oatmeal

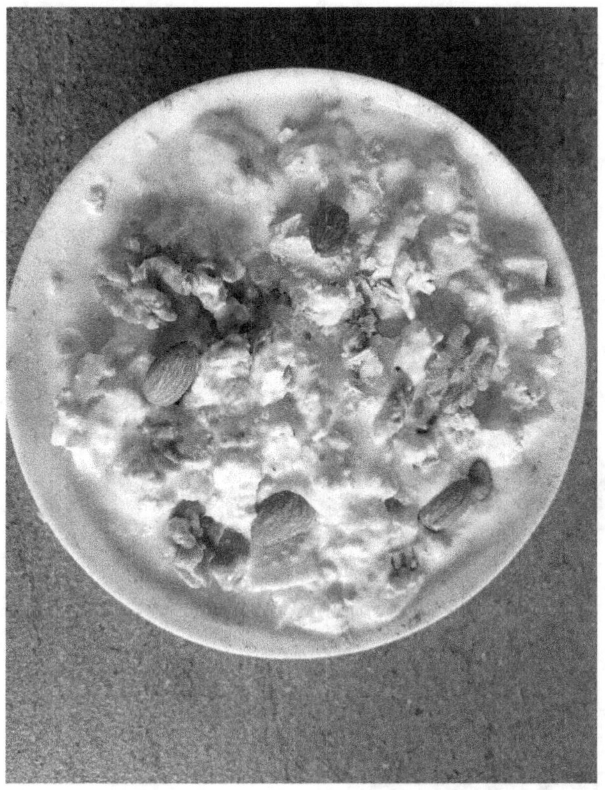

Steps:

1) Take a bowl with handful of Oatmeal
2) Add 250g of low fat yogurt
3) Sliced banana, mix blueberries, blackberries and 1 chopped Apple

4) Add Almond Cinnamon and mix properly

Chapter 4

Yogurt, Cinnamon and Chia seed Parfait

Recipe 3

Ingredients

1: 1 cup coconut milk Yogurt
2: 2 tablespoon Chia seeds
3: 1/4 teaspoon Cinnamon
4: 1/4 cup unsweetened almond milk
5: 2 Tablespoon sliced almonds
6: 3 pieces of dates(chopped)

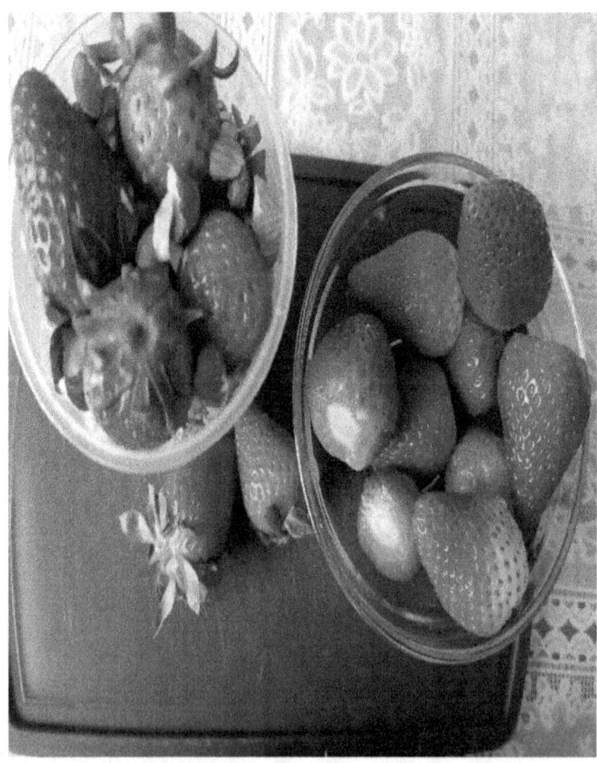

Steps:

1) Combine the almond milk, chia seeds and coconut milk yogurt in a bowl

2) Pour one layer of the mixture into a glass

3) Add the almond and Cinnamon

4) Repeat this process until you have 3 layers

5) Refrigerate the glass for 12 minutes to thicken the Parfait and serve chilled

Chapter 5

Banana Almond Yogurt

Recipe 4

Ingredients:

1: 1/2 Large Banana sliced

2: 1 Tablespoon raw, crunchy, unsalted almond butter

3: 3/4 cup coconut milk yogurt

4: 1 Tablespoon Honey

5: 1/8 teaspoon ground cinnamon

6: 1/2 cup unsalted almonds

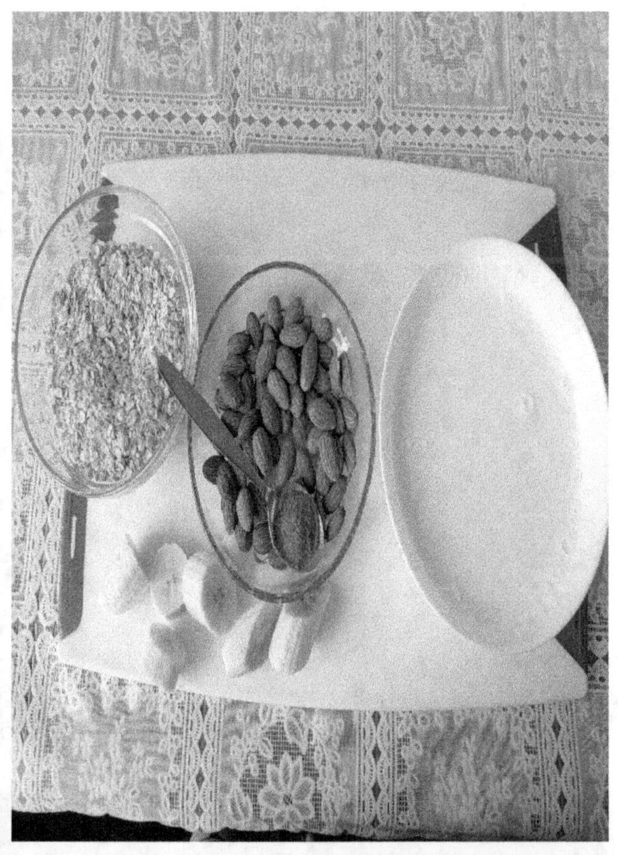

Steps:

1) Soften the almond butter in a microwave for 20 seconds
2) Scop the coconut milk yogurt into a bowl, stir in the almond and banana
3) sprinkle cinnamon on top

Chapter 6

Almond Flour Pancakes

Recipe 5

Ingredients:

1: 1 Cup unsweetened almond milks
2: 3 large eggs
3: 1 1/2 cups almond meal
4: 1/2 teaspoon vanilla essence
5: 1/4 teaspoon baking powder
6: Pinch of salt

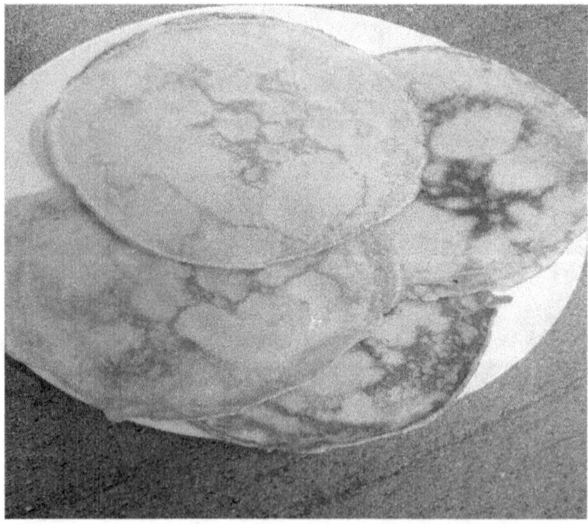

Steps:

1) Mix the dry ingredients in a larger bowl
2) Mix the almond milk eggs and vanilla in a small bowl
3) Add the wet ingredients to the dry ingredient, mixing well until you achieve a smoo
consistency

Heat a grill pan to medium, heat and coat it with olive oil spray
Use a ladle to pour batter onto the pan, and cook the pancakes 2-3 minutes
Flip the pancakes when they begin to bubble on top and continue cooking for a
rther minute
Remove from the heat and stalk on a covered plate until all the pancakes have been
oled
Serve right away

Chapter 7

Green Bean Stir-Fry

Recipe 6

Ingredients:

1 1/2 tablespoon vegetable broth
1/2 tablespoon sesame oil
1/2 tablespoon coconut aminos sauce
1/4 clove garlic minced
1/4 pound green bean, trimmed
1/4 tablespoon toasted sesame seeds

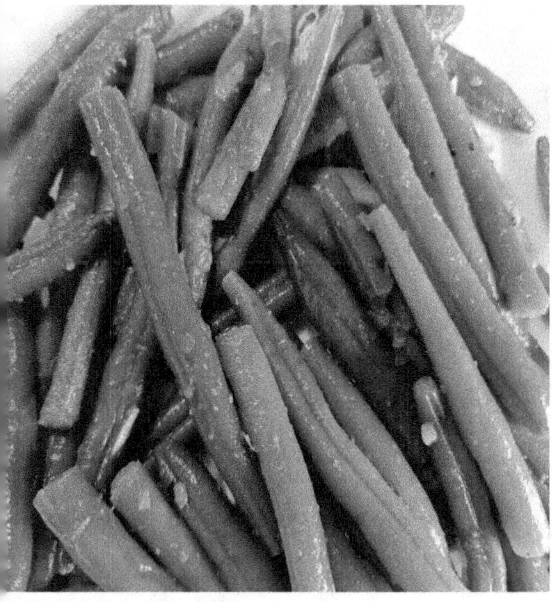

Steps:

1) Combine the coconut aminos and the vegetable broth in a bowl and mix vigorous
2) Heat a skillet for 60 seconds. Add sesame oil, allowing it to coat the bottom of the
pan
3) Add green beans, stir-frying for 5 minutes
4) Add the vegetable broth mixture, garlic and ginger and stir-fry for 1 minute
5) Cover the skillet, cooking for 2 minutes
6) Remove the cover and continue cooking until there is no liquid left in the skillet
7) Sprinkle with sesame seeds to serve

Chapter 8

SUPER LUNCHES

Lemon and Tarragon-Marinated Salmon

Recipe 7

Ingredients:

1: 1/8 teaspoon coarse salt
2: 1/8 teaspoon freshly ground pepper
3: 1/8 cup fresh lemon juice
4) 1/4 tablespoon extra virgin olive oil
5) 1/4 tablespoon fresh tarragon
6) 1 Salmon fillet
7) Sliced lemon to garnish

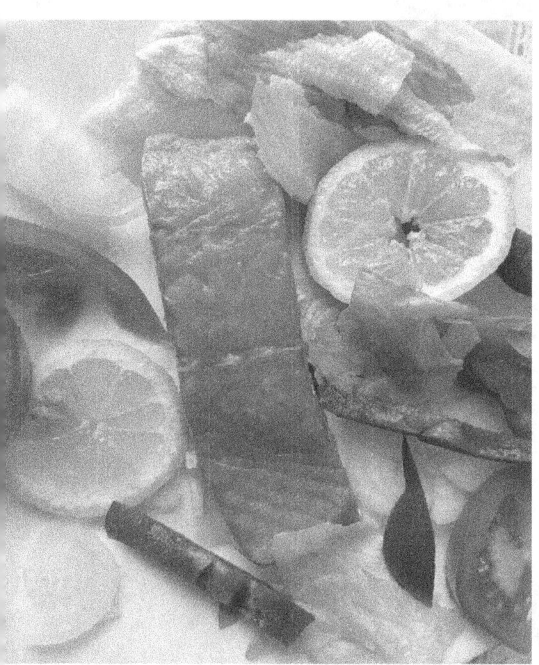

ps:

to make the marinade, combine all ingredients except the salmon in a dish, mixing
l
Add the salmon filet, and coat it liberally, cover and refrigerate for 30 minutes
Remove the filet from the marinade, and place on a grill coated with a non- stick olive
spray over a medium heat
Grill for 10 minutes
Garnish with a slice of lemon

hapter 9

range Sauce with Asparagus

cipe 8

redients:

tablespoon fresh orange juice
tablespoon coconut oil
/2 tablespoon finely grated orange rind
/2- pound fresh asparagus spears tough ends removed

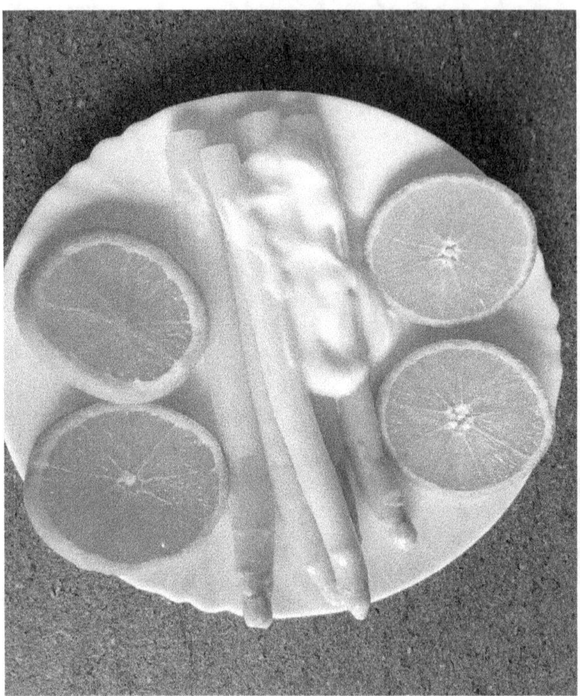

Steps:

1) To make the orange sauce mix the coconut oil, orange juice and orange rind in a small saucepan over a medium heat cook for 4-6 minutes
2) Boil salted water in a large skillet. Add asparagus and blanch for 1-2 minutes u crisp
3) Transfer asparagus to a colander,rinsing thoroughly in cold water. Dry with a pa towel
4) Drizzle orange juice over asparagus to serve

Chapter 10

Green Beans with Almond

Recipe 9

Ingredients

1: 1 tablespoon coconut oil
2: 1/4 pound green beans, trimmed
3: 1/8 cup sliced almonds
4: 1/8 teaspoon coarse salt

5: teaspoon freshly ground pepper

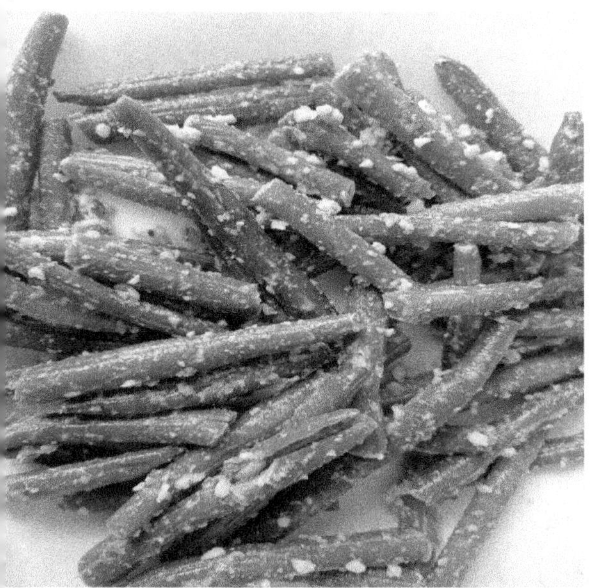

Steps:

1) Boil salted water in a large saucepan over high heat
2) Add green beans and cook for 6 minutes, until crisp. Transfer green beans to a colander   and rinse with cold water. Dry with a paper towel
3) Melt coconut oil in a large skillet over medium heat
4) Add almonds, salt and pepper and saute for 2 minute stirring frequently
5) Add green beans and saute for 2 minutes, stirring frequently

Chapter 11

Tuna Salat

Recipe 10

Ingredients:

1: 1/4 cup chopped Roma tomato
2: 1/4 cup chopped celery
3: 1/2 jalapeno chile pepper, seeded and chopped
4: 1/4 cup chopped red onion
5: 2 (170g) cans albacore tuna in water, no salt added, drained
6: 1 teaspoon brown mustard

7: 3 tablespoon coconut milk yogurt
8: 1/8 teaspoon cracked black pepper
9: 1 small avocado, thinly sliced

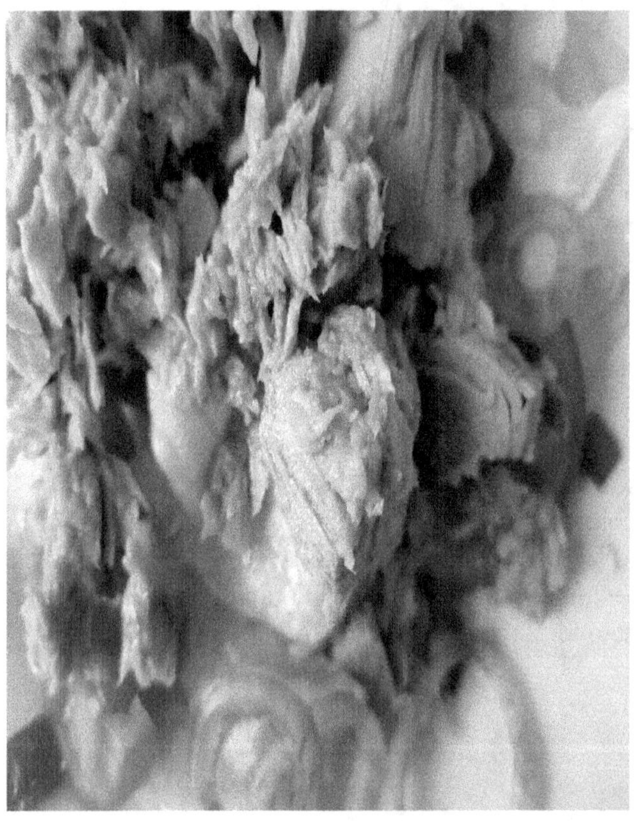

Steps:

1) In a medium bowl, combine the celery, chile pepper, tomato and onion
2) Mix in the tuna, mustard, yogurt, and pepper until well combined
3) Top the salad with avocado slices, and serve

Chapter 12

DELICIOUS DINNERS

Hamburger Curry

Recipe 11

Ingredients:

1/2- pound ground beef
1/4 cup chopped onion
1/2 teaspoon curry powder
4 ounce (114g) tomato sauce
1 clove garlic
1/4 cup water
1 teaspoon lemon juice
1/4 head cauliflower

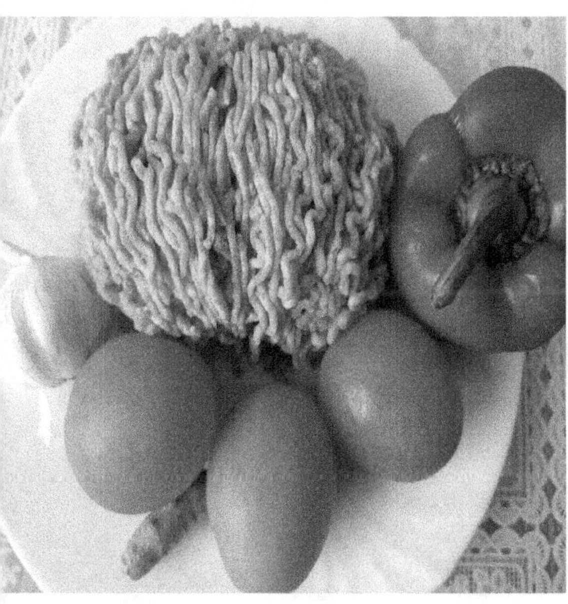

Steps:

Brown the ground beef in a skillet with medium heat
Pour off the fat and add in the onions, curry, garlic, tomato sauce and water
Cover, turn down the heat and allow to simmer for 30 more minutes then add the
lemon juice and let it simmer for 5 more minutes

4) Place the cauliflower in a food processor and shred thoroughly place in a microwavable casserole dish and microwave for 5 minutes on high with a tablespoon water
5) Serve the curry over the cauli- rice

Chapter 13

Baked sole in Creamy Curry Sauce

Recipe 12

Ingredients:

1: 1/2 cup coconut milk yogurt
2: 1/4 cup canned coconut milk
3: 1/2 tablespoon lemon juice
4 1/2 teaspoon Curry powder
5: 1-pound sole filets

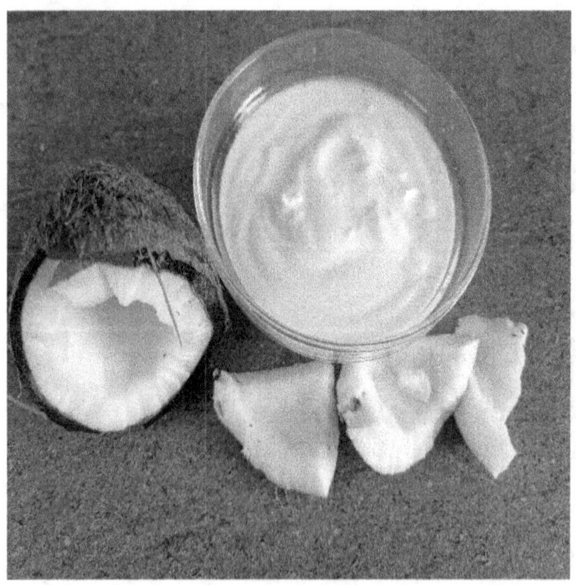

Steps:

1) To make the sauce, mix everything except the sole filets
2) Spray an 8" x 8" baking dish with non-stick cooking spray

Spread the filets with some sauce, rolling them up and down to thoroughly coat them,
ce in the baking dish
Spoon the rest of the sauce over and around the dish
Bake at 350 degrees F for 30 minute

hapter 14

an- Barbecued Sea Bass

ecipe 13

redients:

1/2-pound sea bass filet
1 tablespoon classic barbeque rub
2 slices bacon
1 tablespoon lemon juice

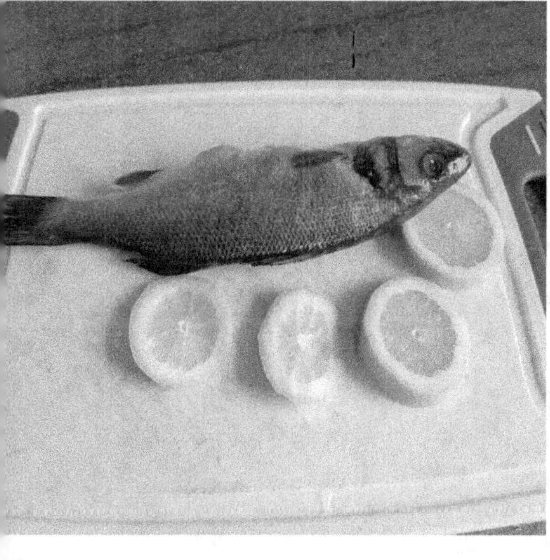

eps:

Sprinkle both sides od the filet with the Barbecue rub
Spray a large skillet with non-stick cooking spray and place over a low heat
Using scissors to cut small portions of bacon directly into the skillet
After 2 minutes, add the fish filets
After 4 minutes, flip the fish over stirring the bacon cook for a further 4 minutes
Take the filets off the heat and put on a serving plate

7) Top with the browned bacon and pour on the lemon juice

Chapter 15

Coconut-Fried Tilapia

Recipe 14

Ingredients:

1: 2 tablespoons coconut oil
2: 1/2 cup shredded coconut
3: 1/2- pound tilapia filets
4: juice and zest of 1 lemon
5: salt and pepper to taste
6: Paprika to taste

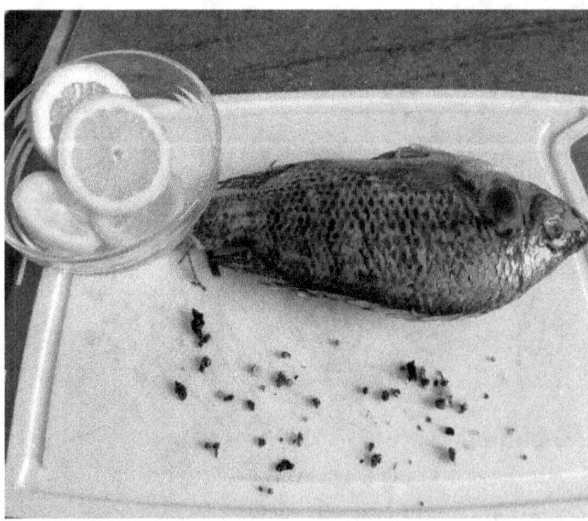

Steps:

1) Preheat the oven to 450 degrees F. Put coconut oil in a baking dish and place in
hot oven until it is melted

Stirr in the coconut and bake for another 5 minutes
Reduce heat to 400 degrees F. Place the fish in the hot oil and bake for 15 minutes
Turn the filets and baste with the pan juice
Sprinkle the filet with lemon juice, lemon zest, salt,pepper and paprika
Bake for 5 more minutes

Chapter 16

Chile Con Carne

Recipe 15

Ingredients:

1/2-Pound lemon ground beef
1/2 medium yellow onion, diced
1 tablespoon chile powder
1/2 412g can stewed tomatoes
1/2 teaspoon salt
1/4 teaspoon cumin
1/4 teaspoon red pepper
1 bay leaf
1 whole clove garlic

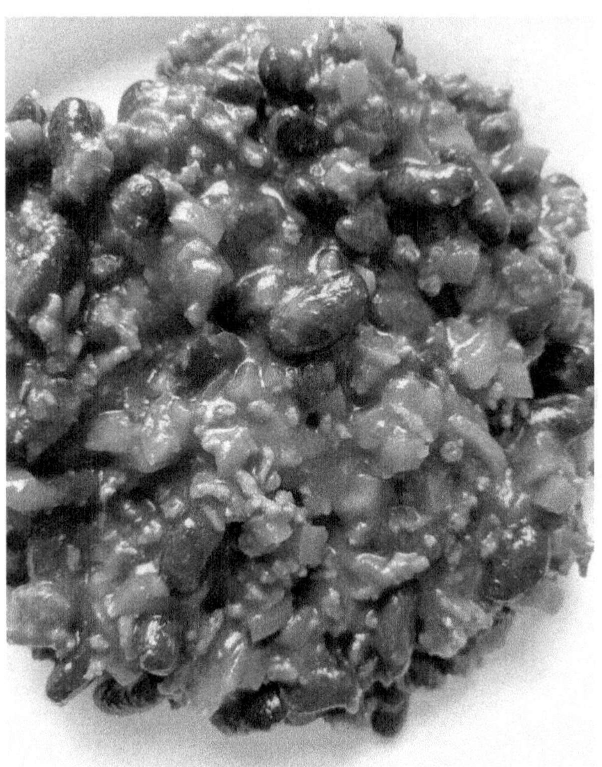

Steps:

1) Brown the ground beef in a saucepan on a medium heat-Drain off excess fat
2) Add the remaining ingredients. Cover and simmer on a low heat for 1 hour che
after 30 minutes and add water if needed
3) Remove bay leaf serve warm with diced onion as toppings

Chapter 17

Fried eggs with Spinach and Olive

Recipe 16

Ingredients:

1: 4 pieces of eggs
2: Salt to taste
3: 1 tablespoon of olive oil
4: Pepper to taste
5: Spinach

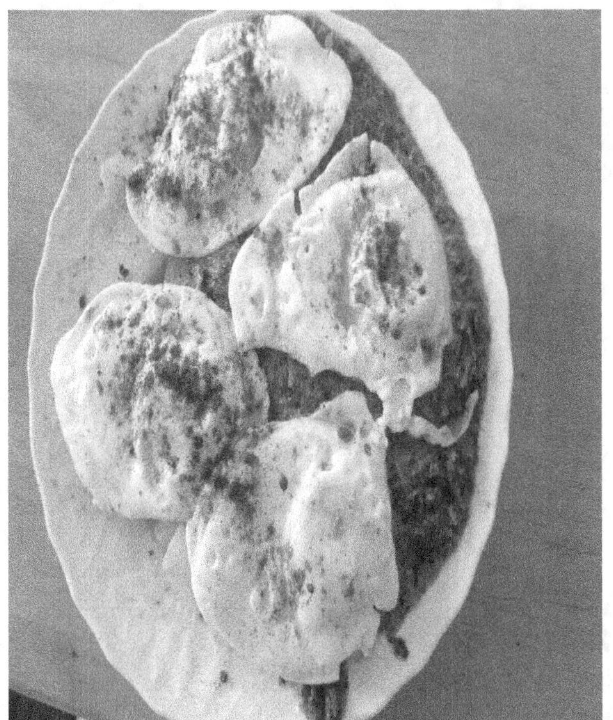

Steps:

1) Break the eggs in bowl
2) Chopped the spinach to pieces
3) Add the spinach to the bowl. Mix properly and some and pepper to taste
4) Heat up the pan add 1 tablespoon of olive oil and fry
5) Serve with some olive

Chapter 18

Pomegranate Salad

Recipe 17

Ingredients:

1: 4 cups arugula
2: 1 large avocado, pitted, peeled and chopped
3: 1/2 cup thinly sliced Anjou pears, thinly sliced
4: 1/2 cup thinly sliced fennel
5: 1/4 cup pomegranate seeds

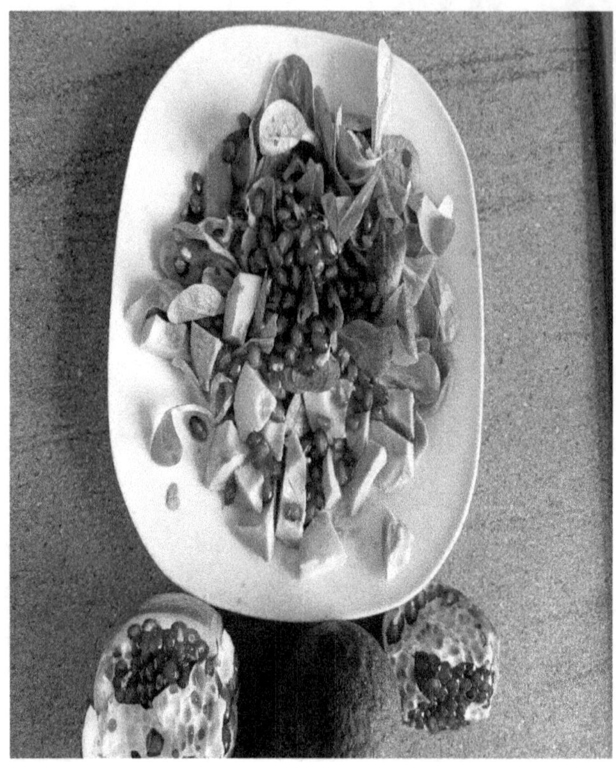

Steps:

1) In a large bowl combine all the ingredients, adding the pomegranate seeds la
2) Toss well, and serve with olive oil and vinegar dressing

Chapter 19

Bell pepper salad

Recipe 18

Ingredients:

Per serving

1: 1/2 red bell pepper:-- Energy 12 Kcal
2: 1/2 yellow bell pepper: --Total Fat 0g
3: 1 tomato (chopped :-- Saturated Fat 0g

4: 1/2 cucumber (chopped & peeled) :--Protein 0 g

5: Low sodium salt to taste:-- Carbohydrate 2.5g

6: 1/2 green bell pepper:-- Dietary Fiber 0,5 g

7: Oregano to taste: Sugar 0g

8: Chili Flakes to taste: –Sodium 1000 mg

9: 2 teaspoon lemon juice:--Cholesterol 0mg

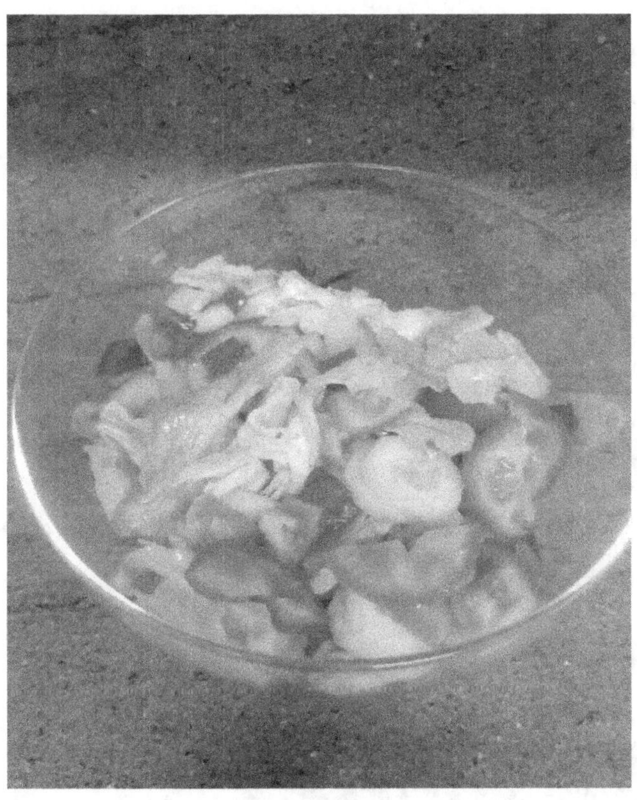

Chapter 20

Broccoli High Protein Salad

Recipe 19

Ingredients:

1. 1 cucumber sliced in half ring form
2. 1 Radish sliced in half ring form
3. 1 tomato sliced
4. 1 onion sliced
5. Lettuce leaf sliced
6 1/3 Bell pepper red and yellow both sliced
7. broccoli sliced and steam for 3- 4 minutes
8. roasted peanuts and boiled kidney beans
9. white boiled chana
10. 100 g paneer

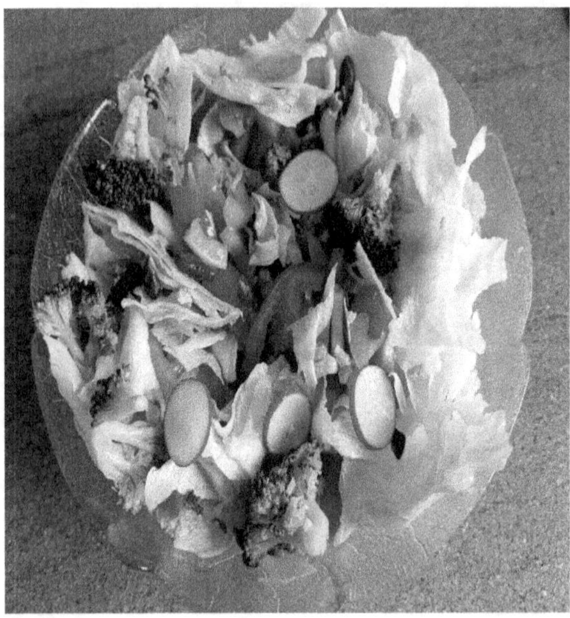

Steps:

1) Mix all in a bowl and add 2 - 3 tablespoons of lemon juice, 1/2 teaspoon of salt .
2) Mix in a small bowl 2 tablespoons of olive oil with 1 tablespoon of black pepper a
add to the mix.

Add some fresh coriander and last chat masala powder and roasted cumins powder
ix properly and serve.

or more nutrition guides visit us at: https://superfoods.pages.dev/#aff=IsaacAustin

Chapter 21

REFRESHING DRINKS, TIPS AND TRICKS

Beetroot juice

Recipe 20

ngredients:

2 pieces beetroot
2 pieces carrots
2 pieces of apple
1 lime/ lemon
10g of ginger

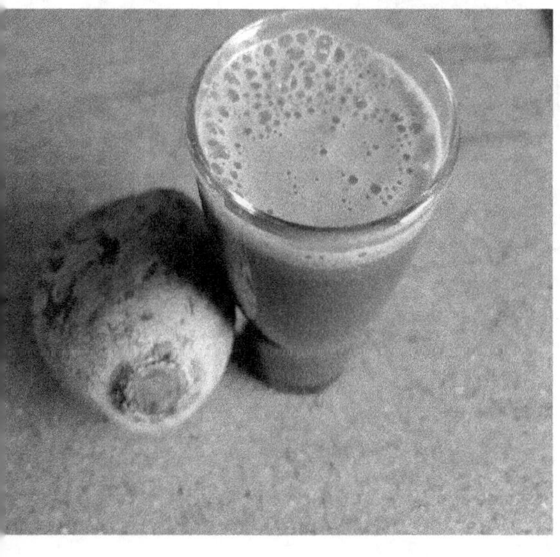

Steps:

wash and scrape carrots, and beetroot properly with water

2) Cut the apple and ginger, peel the ginger middle pieces
3) Peel the lemon/lime, remove the seeds
4) Juice them / blend then strain it and serve fresh

Chapter 22

Pomegranate Juice

Recipe 21

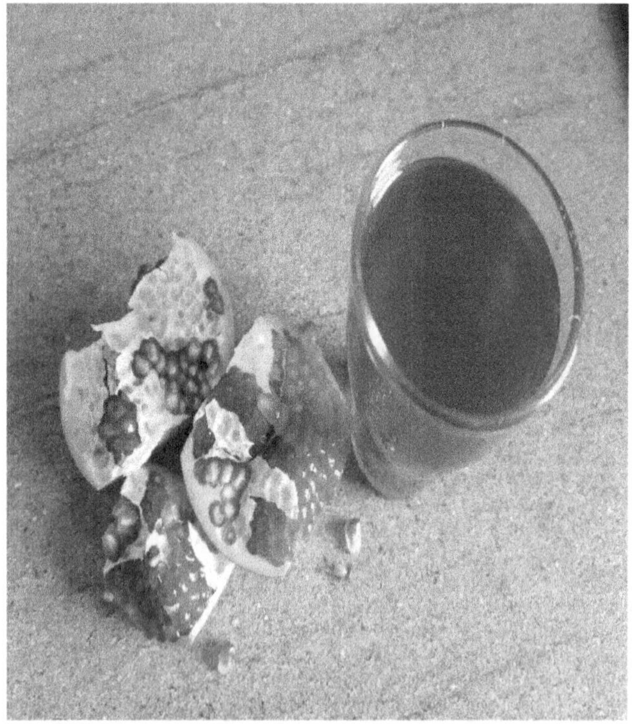

4 Pieces Pomegranate

Watermelon juice with lime/Lemon

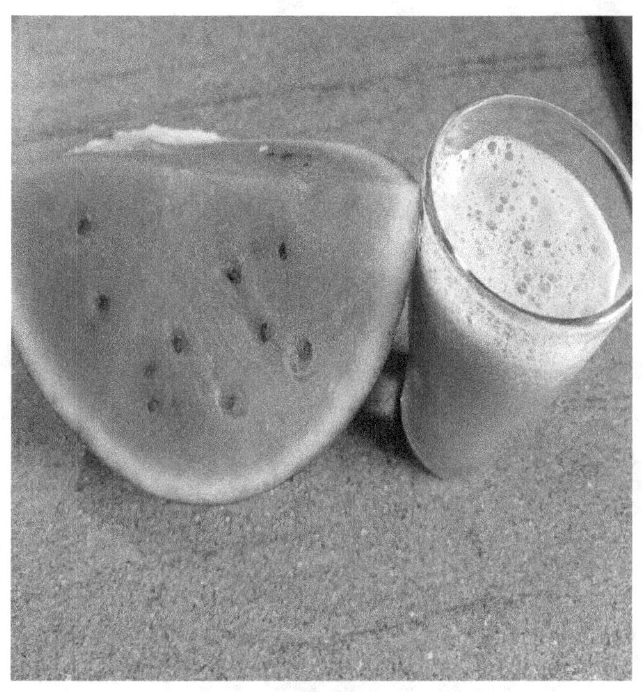

Steps:

Chopped some pieces of watermelon.
Blend and strain the watermelon
Add 1 pieces of lime / lemon

Watermelon, beetroot and Carrot juice

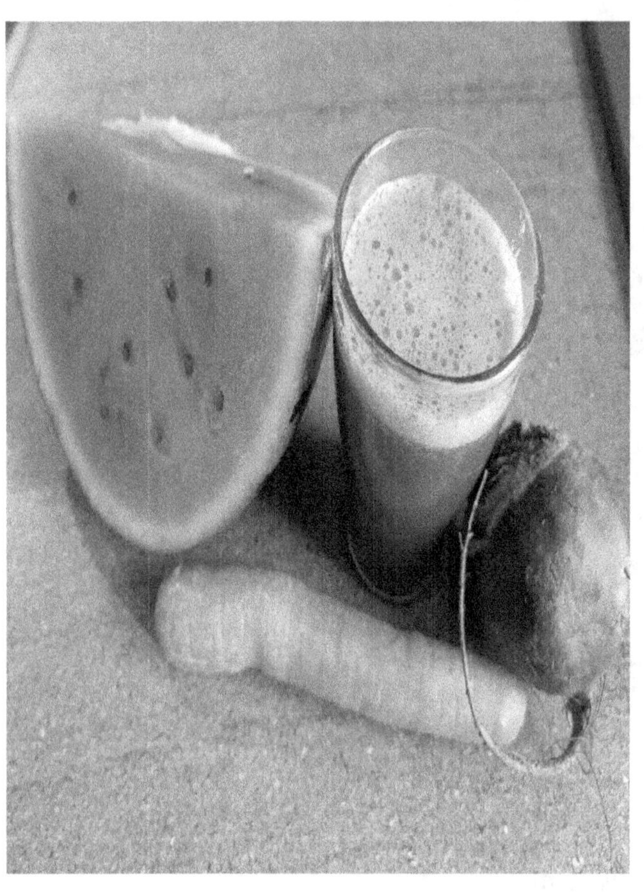

Watermelon, Ginger and beetroot juice

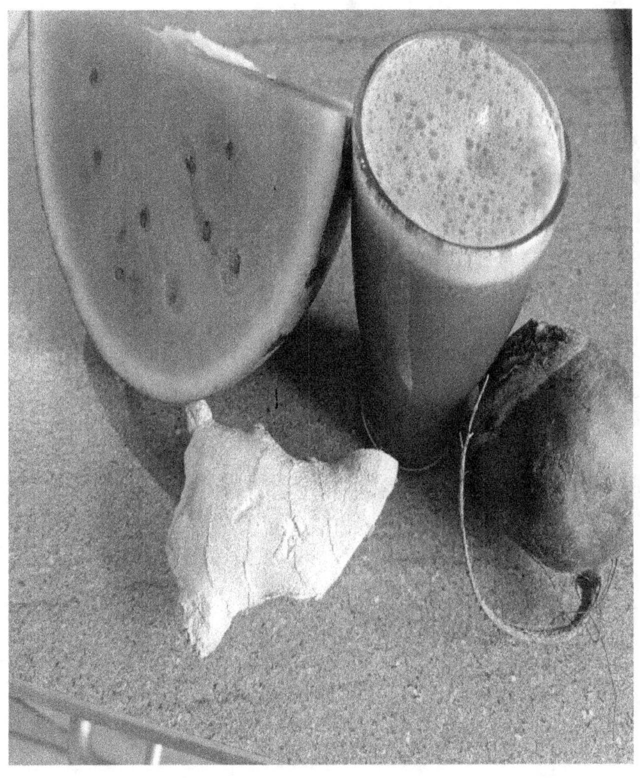

Watermelon, Ginger and beetroot juice(best for men)

Watermelon and strawberries juice

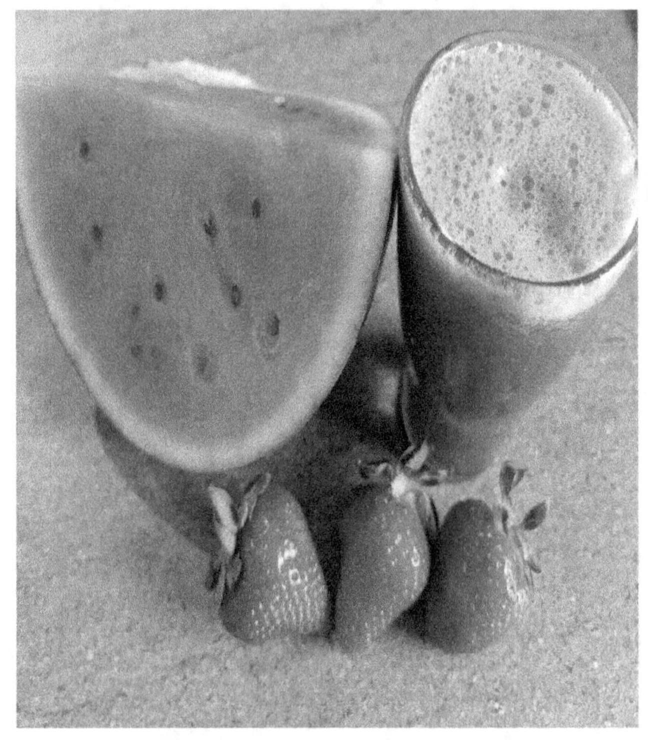

Watermelon and strawberries juice

Turmeric Drink

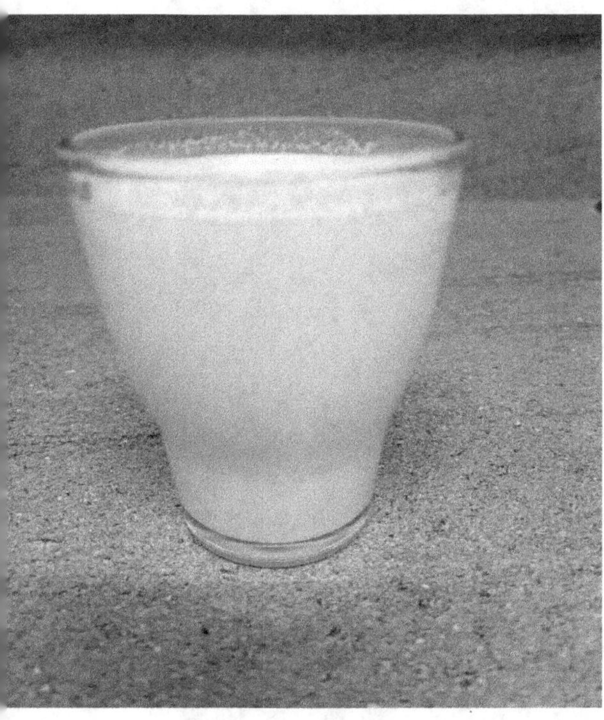

2 teaspoon of Turmeric in a glass of warm Almond milk with a teaspoon honey

Celery juice

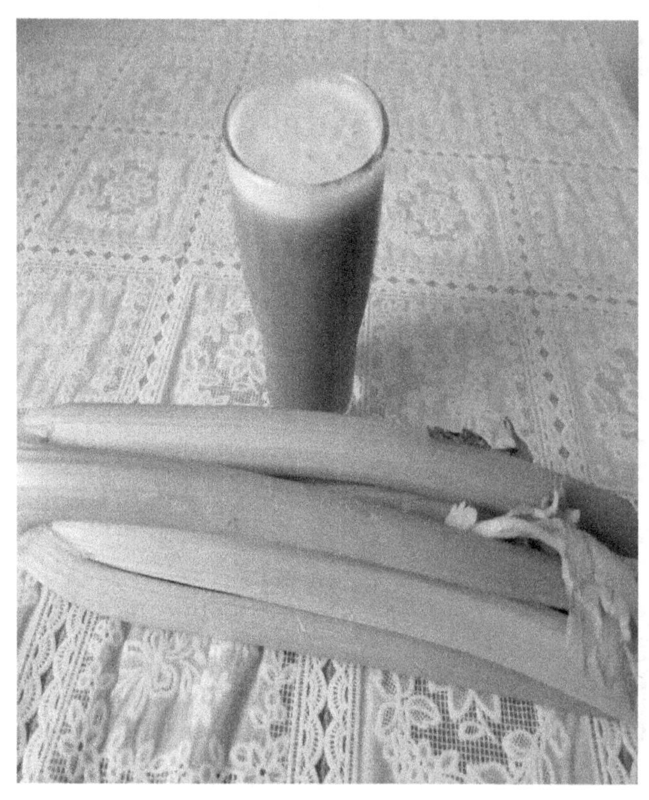

Figs in olive oil

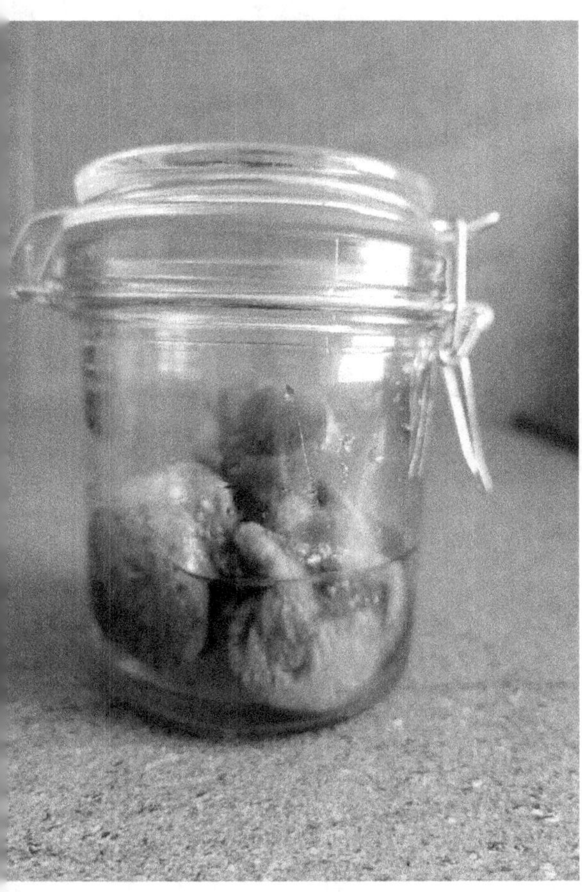

gs in olive oil, eat 3 pieces in the morning before breakfast

Conclusion

ou probably know by now that eating healthy and exercising can lower your blood
essure naturally without having to take any pills (seek your doctor advice).
se low sodium salt
void processed foods / packaged foods

or more healthy juicing visit.https://healthy-juicing.pages.dev/#aff=IsaacAustin

at healthy, live healthy

www.ingramcontent.com/pod-product-compliance
Lightning Source LLC
Chambersburg PA
CBHW060906260726
48661CB00008B/3491